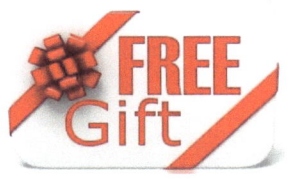

Want Priority Access to FREE eBooks Additional Materials for this Book?

As we release NEW eBooks, we offer them for FREE for a limited time. You will be the FIRST one to know when they are FREE. Join 1000's of insiders who are getting access to FREE Kindle book promotions weekly.

Click HERE for FREE additional material and FREE eBooks-
www.rictamilypublishing.com

TABLE OF CONTENTS

PILATES

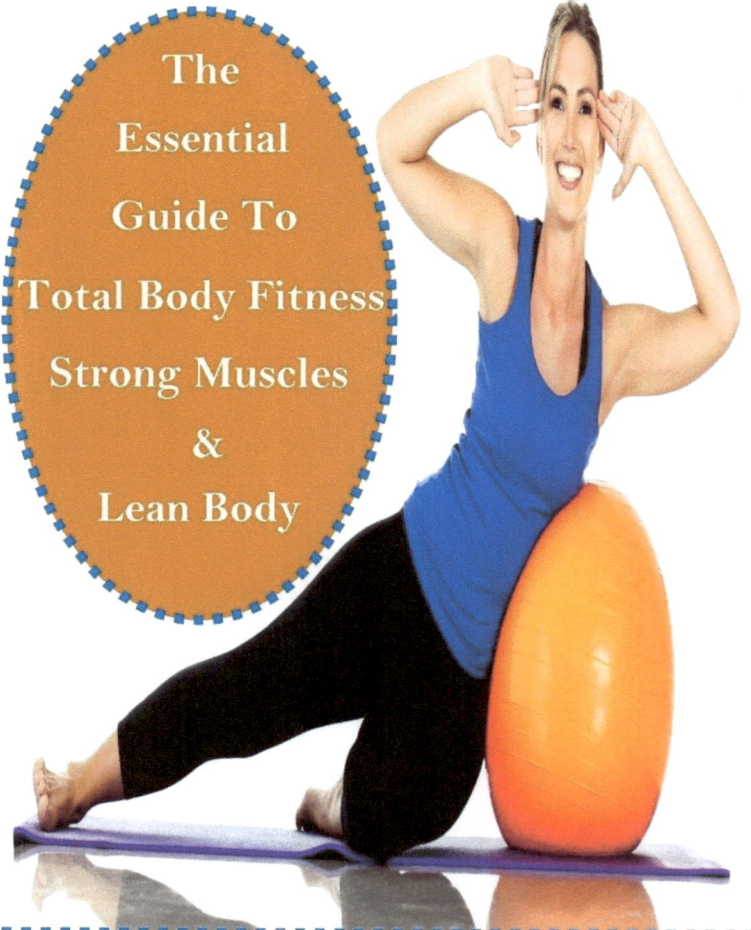

The
Essential
Guide To
Total Body Fitness
Strong Muscles
&
Lean Body

Tammi Diamond

INTRODUCTION

I want to thank you and congratulate you for downloading the book *"PILATES FOR BEGINNERS: The Essential Guide to Total Body Fitness, Strong Muscles and Lean Body"*.

This book contains proven steps and strategies on how to achieve total body conditioning, strong muscles and lean body. By reading this book, you will have a deeper understanding of what Pilates is all about, and the main points and ideas that would truly condition our body achieve total body fitness, strong muscles and lean body.

Here's an inescapable fact: you will need more than knowledge of a few poses and exercises to achieve what Pilates truly strives for.

If you do not develop your understanding of what Pilates is and the teachings that it imparts, even the most difficult poses and exercises will not attain for your total body fitness.

It's time for you to become an amazing student of Pilates, one that understands this amazing workout exercise.

CHAPTER 1
Getting to Know Pilates

There are many forms of exercise that are popular nowadays. These include yoga, Tai Chi, Chi-gong and Pilates. In this book, we will discover more about Pilates, its benefits and the forms of exercise that can be used in maintaining a healthy body with lean and developed muscles.

Pilates and its History

This is a method of conditioning the body invented by Joseph Pilates. It is a technique of having the body and mind fuse, leading to an improvement in posture, strength, flexibility and an overall change in how a person feels about his or her body.

This program was originally designed as a rehabilitation program for the veterans of World War I as controlling or mat work. The developer designed it after his apprenticeship and study of Ancient Roman and Greek physical regimens, Zen and Yoga. Precise movements were formed because of his belief in the connection between mind and body. The movements are focused on the form and control of the entire body. Through its principles, a person experiences the transformation of the body as a whole.

The difference between other exercises and Pilates is that it develops multiple groups of muscles simultaneously. Joseph Pilates believed that building a strong core or powerhouse was essential. This core is comprised of the muscles under the shoulder blades, those surrounding the rib cage and down to the gates and hips.

The Core

The integration of the trunk, pelvis and shoulder girdle is the way to achieve core control. The techniques involved in Pilates pave the way to developing physical energy from the core to manifest the movements of the limbs. All movements are focused on muscle control. Each movement was created for a certain purpose; therefore, each is a contributor to the success as a whole.

The exercises not only develop weak muscles, but enhance the elasticity of the muscles as well as the balance of the body.

Materials

Most of the movements under the Pilates are mat exercises, meaning they are performed on the ground. However, there are numerous Pilate's machines that can aid in exercising. The difference is, in mat works, your own body weights acts as the resistance. On the other hand, machines facilitate increased intensity because of the additional resistance from the spring.

CHAPTER 2
Pilates Principles

In order to keep track of obtaining certain objectives, principles must be followed. The principles were designed to be followed and to guide the performance of each exercise.

The Six Principles of Pilates

There are over 500 exercises related to Pilates and each exercise was rooted from the following principles:

Centering. The center of the core is the most important part of the body. It is also the area of focus in Pilate's exercises. It was believed that the energy needed to do the exercises correctly comes from the core center. The energy flows outside the body and manifests in the movements of the limbs. Through the core center, a strong foundation and stability can be maintained.

Breathing. One of the most important principles knows how to breathe with precision, concentration and control. The developer believed that in order to awaken the cells in our body, blood circulation is necessary. In order to have a good blood circulation, oxygen must be distributed throughout the body and wastes shall be eliminated.

The developer also believed that the proper oxygenation of the muscles shall be achieved through thorough and full inhalation and exhalation. Inhalation requires the maintenance of engagement while exhalation requires the engagement of pelvic muscles, together with the abdomen and the rib cage.

Precision. The focus of the movements in Pilates requires precision. The intrinsic value of each movement and their purpose are forsaken if there is no precision. This shall be the second nature of each practitioner of Pilates.

Concentration. Quality is more important than quantity. When doing a precise movement, one must have an effective concentration. By concentrating, you will become aware of how your body feels. It is also important that your mind and body act as one to produce precise movements.

Control. The purpose of every movement is to enhance muscle control. Thus, doing sloppy and uncontrolled movements are not effective in achieving such purpose. Work becomes more efficient when there is control and balance in the body.

Flow. Efficiency shall be continuous. The transitions between exercises must be smooth. This will improve stamina and strength. This will also allow the body to master safe and efficient movements.

CHAPTER 3
Why do Men and Women Practice Pilates?

To get involved in an exercise program means that you have a goal. These goals will help endure the pain. Each person definitely has driving force that will help them achieve their wants or needs.

Why do men practice Pilates?

There are many reasons for doing Pilates; however, these are the most common ones.

Building strength and power.

The Pilates focus is promoting core strength and letting it flow outward to the limbs. By using a core strength, performance is maximized and power is built. The practitioner of Pilates found it easy to perform explosive movements more efficiently. The strong foundation of strength and power is core stability.

Developing neglected muscles. We cannot deny the fact that most of the muscles in the body are undeveloped. The muscles that we need in our daily activities, such as those in the arms and legs, are stronger than other muscles. In doing Pilates, the movements help to divert effort from primary muscles and tone the neglected ones. The agonist muscles, supporting muscles, become more developed while doing Pilates.

Enhancing Flexibility. Flexibility is often based on muscle mass. More muscle masses tend to decrease flexibility. However, by practicing Pilates, flexibility is enhanced. This will lead to a lower chance of acquiring muscles strains and injuries.

Improved Stamina. Men who work jobs that require great stamina can benefit from Pilates. Studies have shown that middle aged men who practice Pilates have significantly increased upper-body and abdominal strength and endurance.

Why do women practice Pilates?

While men do Pilates for physical advancement, most women do this for health, style and beauty. The following are the most common reasons women do Pilates.

Help in the preparation for pregnancy. For a pregnant woman, Pilates will be of great help in strengthening the pelvic floor, back and tummy muscles without giving stress to other joints. There are several Pilates classes conducted especially for pregnant women. The benefit is increased function in the muscles that may give rise to problems during pregnancy.

Pilates also promotes balance. This will help you walk and stand properly without tripping or falling due to your baby bump. It also helps in learning proper breathing that is necessary in labor.

Full body sculpting. The most common workout for women focuses on sole cardiovascular exercises. However, this type of workout does not eliminate excessive calories in the body. The true exercise must be a combination of strength enhancement and cardiovascular endurance.

Pilates can give you a full body workout, which is a must in sculpting your body. You might feel that your whole body is at sore when you first take classes, but this will eventually shape up your body.

CHAPTER 4
Workouts for Beginners

In every engagement, you must start with the basics. This will help your body to adopt in the movements. This will help lessen the risk of injury or strain.

The Warm Up

1. *Starting Position - Constructive Rest - Neutral Spine*

   - This will be the first position to perform prior to other fundamental exercises.

   - You must lie on your back, arms by your side. Bend your knees with feet flat on the floor about a hip distance apart. Inhale and exhale. Use your ABS to press your spine into the floor.

2. *Head nod*

   - This is an extension to obtain a lengthened spine. This is an essential part of numerous Pilate's exercises involving articulation of the spine.

   - In performing this, start with the neutral spine position. To lengthen your spine, inhale. Then, tilt your chin towards your chest without removing your head from the mat.

   - Exhale to return to the first position. Repeat the cycle again.

3. *Arms over*

- This focuses on the alignment of the body. This also challenges the torso by lifting the arms overhead. This also enables the enhancement of the shoulder joint range.

- To perform this motion, start with the first position. Inhale as you bring your hands up to the ceiling. Exhale as you rest your arms on the floor behind you.

- Repeat the cycle.

Basic Movements for Beginners

1. *Pilates Hundreds*

- To start, lie on your back and bend your knees with your feet flat on the floor. Your arms should be at your side, palms down. Tilt your hips to contract your ABS, pushing down your lower back against the mat. Simultaneously, lift your head, neck, and shoulder blades off the floor. Continue while inhaling and exhaling slowly.

- Lastly, pump your arms in an up and down motion by your sides, palms facing the floor. This should be done in a pressing motion.

2. *Pilates Kneeling Rear Leg Raises*

- Start on knees and elbows on the mat, evenly distributing your weight. Your knees should be properly placed directly under your hip joints. Also, your elbows shall be directly under your shoulder sockets. Pull your belly button toward your spine.

- Extend one leg. Your toes shall not touch the ground. Lift your leg as high as you can, this will make your back arch.

- Switch legs and repeat.

CHAPTER 5
Moves for Burning Calories

These are the movements used by women who want to achieve their desired body. These steps enable them to burn excessive calories in the body.

Swimming

The first step is to lie on your stomach with pubis firmly anchored in the mat, forehead down and inner thighs tightly pressed together. Your arms should be stretched forward as far as possible with the palms down and toes pointed. In a count of one, lift altogether your arms, chest, head and legs and hold.

Inhale and exhale normally while alternately lifting your arms and legs without touching the ground. Occasionally lift higher and reach longer for progress.

Crisscross

To start, lie on your back with your hands behind your lifted head, palm over another. Your knees should be bent tightly into your chest. As you inhale slowly, twist your torso to the left until your right elbow touches your left knee. Straighten your right leg and hold it a few inches above the mat. Exhale and do the same procedure on the other side.

Six sets of twists are recommended.

Jogging Knees with Heel Ups

Your elbows shall be pinned to your sides and your ABS shall be pulled in and up as you begin lifting your knees in a hip height. After approximately 8 knee lifts, begin kicking your bottom using your heels. After that kicks, you have the option to continue another set or move on to the next exercise.

Leg Pull

To begin, sit tall and extend your legs straight, squeezing them tightly together. Your feet should be pointed. Rest your palms on the edge of the mat behind you with your fingers pointing inward. Put the pressure on your hands as you elevate your hips. Make your body look like a diagonal line from head to heels.

Inhale as you lift your right leg as high as possible without losing your balance. Exhale as you control your feet as they return to the mat.

Switch legs and repeat the steps.

CHAPTER 6

Pilates Moves for a Flat Stomach

Every woman wants good posture and a flat stomach. Here are some moves that will result in a flat stomach.

Saw

To perform this exercise, sit tall with your back straight and waist lengthened. Your arms should be opened straight out to your sides at shoulder level and form a "crack- a - walnut" figure between your shoulder blades. Your legs are open wider than your shoulders, together with a flexed foot from the ankles and an anchored bottom of the mat.

Inhale while you rotate your trunk to your left and round over your left knee, as you press your right hand against the out edge of your left foot. Lift your arm back as high as possible. Exhale as you slide your right hand to the outside of the left foot in sawing motions as you draw back, creating diagonal opposition for your ABS.

Inhale as you return to the first position and perform three sets.

Double-Leg Stretch

Hug both your knees into your chest with your head forward, lifted and your elbows wide.

Control your inhalation as you reach your legs forward and arms in backward position, each stretching in opposition, which draws your abdomen in deeply to support your spine. Slowly exhale as you return to the first position, with the knees hugged to chest. Expand your diaphragm to allow air to enter your lungs.

Repeat this six times.

Corkscrew

Lie on your back with your arms by your sides. Squeeze your legs tightly together.

As lift your legs overhead, inhale slowly. This will make you roll back until you balance yourself in the middle of your shoulder blades and the back of your arms.

Point your toes while you control your exhalation as you roll back to your spine, your body slightly leaning to the right. Circle your legs to the left as you inhale slowly, as you roll up to your left side. Scoop your ABS and lift your bottom. Shift directions and complete three sets.

CHAPTER 7
Pilates for Larger People

Women are conscious about their bodies; however, many women who are heavy, are comfortable with their weight. Another plus-size women and men are working to lose weight and need a place to start. The following exercises are appropriate for the heavier population.

The Dart

Lie face down on the mat with legs and feet together. Place your arms at your sides and relax your shoulders.

Inhale deeply through your nostrils, and breathe towards the back of your nostrils. Remember to exhale through your mouth. This exercise requires 4 breaths.

Inhale as you open your chest and squeeze shoulders back. Exhale as you reach your hands towards your feet, simultaneously ending your upper body above the floor.

Inhale as you hold the position and lengthen your head and feet in opposite ways. Exhale as you return to your original position.

Pull Down

Grab your exercise band and hold it in place where you feel sufficient tension. Reach your arms over your head with your elbows slightly bent. After this, recheck the tension.

Inhale deeply through your nostrils, and breathe towards the back of your nostrils. Remember to exhale through your mouth. This exercise requires 4 breaths.

In preparing, you must inhale. Exhale as you pull down in front your head as you extend your upper body above the mat. Inhale as you hold this position as you lengthen your head and feet in opposite directions. Exhale as you return.

In performing this, you must keep an eye on your neck and shoulder alignment.

CHAPTER 8
Pilates for a 6-Pack

Male physique can potentially include a six- pack ABS. There are Pilates moves recommended to obtain and maintain six- pack.

Pelvic Bridge or Pelvic Curl

This exercise is often used a warm- up for abdominal muscles and the spine. It also develops the coordination of breathing and movement and promotes the lower body muscles.

Duration is 5 minutes.

To start, find a neutral spine position.

You must breathe in into your chest, to your belly, and to your pelvic floor. You must breathe out of your pelvic area, belly and chest.

Exhale as you tilt your pelvic involving the abdominal muscles and pull your belly button down towards your spine. Continue this action to press the lower spine using your ABS.

Inhale as you press your feet down, enabling your tail bone to begin to curl towards the ceiling. Raise your hips, then your lower spine and finally, the middle spine. Keep your legs parallel all the time.

Repeat this three to five times.

The Roll-Up Ab Pilates Exercise

Start by lying on your back with extended arms along the floor above your head.

Inhale while squeezing your buttock and inner thighs together. Flex your feet. After this, exhale as you roll up, gesturing your straightened arms beyond you. Stretch your arms forward as you place your fingertips, beyond your toes.

Repeat exercise 10-15 times.

CHAPTER 9

Strengthening the legs and back with Pilates

As we age, our back and leg muscles are the most affected. In order to strengthen them, these are the recommended Pilate exercises.

Back Bow Crossover

To start, lie face down on the mat with your arms and legs extended in a straight line. Place an object like dumbbell on the floor above your head at your arm's length. Place both of hands on the left of the object, allowing your body to arch to the left.

Contract your core muscles as you lift your arms and legs up and above to exaggerate the arch to the right. Lower your hands slowly to the right side of the object and let your hands and feet momentarily touch the ground before making another arch to the opposite side.

Do this repetitively for a period of time.

Pilates Back Bows

Lie face down on the mat and extend your arms above your head.

Inhale while contracting your legs and core. Exhale while lifting your chest and arms up above as high as you can.

Inhale as you lower your body to the ground slowly as your arms and chest briefly touch the ground before repeating the steps. Continue without permitting your core to relax.

Lunges

Stand with one foot in front of the other, wide stance as if each foot is placed on a railroad track. Lower toward the ground by bending the knees and lift back up. Repeat several times on each leg. Whatever your weight may be, it is significant for a single leg. This thigh and butt exercise is a great way to tone the muscles in the legs and build lean muscles.

CHAPTER 10
Pilates - The Claims

The following are the claims relating to Pilates exercises.

Leaner and longer muscles

The flexibility of the muscles is increased, which gives rise to the feeling of a longer muscle. Leaner muscles are part of the output of any activity.

Improved postural issues

Postural improvements do not pertain to height, but rather with the strength of the core and the purposeful lifting of each individual. Posture will improve with strength and consciousness to sitting and standing tall on a consistent basis.

Increased stability, peripheral mobility and core strength

Core strength is tested using a device called EMG or Elctromyograph. One of the studies tested the effects of Pilates in the three superficial core muscles, namely rectus abdominis or the ABS, external oblique's or the sides of the abdomen and rectus femoris or the muscles in legs which are used during sit-ups. Findings confirmed that these muscles were positively enhanced by Pilate's exercises. They gained a higher EMG value compared to the general requirements.

Due to the promotion of flexibility, Pilates exercises results to peripheral mobility or mobility the limbs.

Injury prevention

Building core strength can reduce the likeliness of falls and promotes a faster recovery if a fall is encountered.

Enhancing functional fitness and ease of movements

Functional fitness is defined as how the power, endurance, strength and flexibility that influences your daily living functions. As Pilates makes your muscles stronger, daily functions are improved. Physical chores may be completed with more ease and the likelihood of injury is reduced.

Some other claims

These include: balancing strength and flexibility, heightens body awareness, easy on joints with little or no impact. Pilates can be modified to fit everyone, including rehab patients and elite athletes. Pilates complement other methods of exercise, improves sports performance, and lastly, improves circulation, coordination and balance.

CONCLUSION

Thank you again for downloading this book!

I hope this book was able to help you condition your body and achieve a total body fitness, strong muscles and a lean body.

The next step is to live out the teachings that you have learned through this book, and to share them to all that you meet.

Finally, if you enjoyed this book, please take the time to share your thoughts and post a review on Amazon. It'd be greatly appreciated!

Thank you and good luck!

BODYWEIGHT EXERCISES

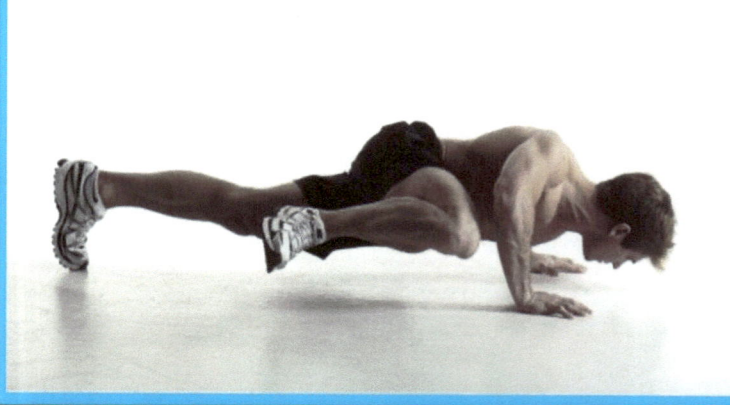

Training to Build Muscle and Lose Fat

Beginner to Advanced Routines

To Strengthen Your Core

Tammi Diamond

INTRODUCTION

I want to thank you and congratulate you for downloading the book, **"Bodyweight Exercises**: *Training to Build Muscles and Lose Fat - Beginner to Advanced Routines to Strengthen Your Core, etc."*

With all the information out there today about what diet to follow, what magic pill to take, you can feel overwhelmed if you need to lose weight. However, anyone who has tried to melt off pounds and get fit knows that trend diets and pills just do not have the longevity that you need to maintain a healthy lifestyle.

It is good old fashioned working out and eating right, which will help you the most. Within the pages of this book you will find surefire workouts that will help strip weight off, tone your core, strengthen your entire cardiovascular system and just feel better. The American medical association speaks highly of doing workouts that strengthen the heart and lungs, while building muscle and this book will help you do it.

There is no doubt that shows like the Biggest Loser and my 600lb. Life has shone a light onto the weight and health problem in the United States today, but these shows also show us first hand the benefits of working out and improving your body. You see contestants go from diabetics with high cholesterol and a huge amount of pill taking daily, too limited or no pills. While that is an extreme example, it holds true in less extreme measures as well and you will find those health building workouts in the pages of this book. Do not wait and see your health getting worse, it is time to get started, get fit and truly enjoy your workout! Whether you need low impact work to protect your joints or prefer doing old fashioned workouts like jumping jacks there is a plan for everyone!

Thanks again for downloading this book, we hope you enjoy it!

CHAPTER 1

The Beginner Core Workout

Starting a new workout routine can be a tough process for anyone who has not done any exercises for an extended period of time. While it would be great if we could all just jump right in and start doing hundreds of burpees, squats and various other exercises right out of the box. The better way is to ease your way back in and build your core and the rest of your body back into prime condition and reclaim your fitness!

In this chapter we will cover the basic routines that you need to get started with core fitness that will lead into full body fitness.

The transverse-abdominals is a muscle that is a deeper a muscle and more often than not it is not given the same attention as other core muscles are. This muscle is the muscle that supports, protects and holds the back up and keeps key organs held where they belong during the workout. While it is often ignored it should not be because of what it protects and because it stabilizes the rectus abdominals and the oblique.

In order to focus on engaging this core muscle you need to make yourself familiar with it start by sucking in your navel toward your spine, while you do that, you will tuck your lower back muscles towards the belly and keep that focus just under your belly button. To truly get to know this muscle you will work it throughout your day both during your gym time and your regular daytime activities. The best way to set a good routine for this is to choose specific times each day to do the described workout. Spend time each day doing the routine in either two to three sets of between 10 and 20 repetitions. Alternatively you can do two to three sets of holding each of your repetitions for between 15 and 45 seconds and once again do two to three sets.

Once you have started work on your rectus abdominus it will be time to move onto your butt muscles also called the glutes. Getting these muscles back to work can be harder than other core groups, but if you focus and put in the work, you can get them working. You will want to stand and place your feet close together, keeping the muscles of your legs firm and tight. While you hold your legs like that press your thighs together and lift to lengthen your posture through the waist. Move your shoulders back and away from your ears and clench your glutes together, while you clench draw the muscles up and hold as firmly as possible. You will hold this clench for between 15 and 45 seconds the longer the better and then relax and repeat the process. While you work these glute muscles you will get the muscles in your lower back moving as well, this is what should happen and an advantage of strengthening your entire core.

The next workout you should start after a solid routine of strengthening routines is the classic sit up or crunch. It might be a very basic exercise but it works and you can do it almost anywhere and with little more than an exercise or yoga mat to keep you comfortable. Once you have laid back you want to place your legs flat on the floor and keep your muscles tight while your legs stay firmly on the floor, you will raise yourself up to fully straight in the back. Ease back down and then repeat. If you find that keeping your legs firmly to the floor is too hard to start you can bend at the knees and keep your feet firmly planted on the floor. With your feet staying planted you pull yourself up keeping your back straight, this is a full sit up. Alternatively you can do a crunch if your core is not strong enough to handle a full sit up without causing back pain. In a crunch you will keep your legs in either the standard or modified position, hold your transverse abdominals tight and bring yourself up to half sitting.

As a beginner, you will want to start with smaller sets to get going, do between one and three sets that include between ten and twelve repetitions. As you get fit and start to feel like you aren't being challenged, you will move to the next level of between three and five sets that include twelve to 16 repetitions and the third level when you have reached a higher level of fitness should include five to seven sets with 16 to 20 repetitions.

You should move upwards through each level when you don't feel challenged. The key to building muscle and toning your body is not to get comfortable and plateau. If you need a challenge that goes beyond the third level in crunches you can add in holding a medicine ball with weight to it through each set. Additionally, you can cut sets out altogether and just do as many sit-ups and or crunches as possible, when you stop write down the number that you did in a workout notebook so that next time you can increase the amount that you do. Continuing you challenge yourself by adding more crunches and sit ups and a heavier medicine ball as you improve will ensure that you get a strong core and a set of six pack abs.

Planking is the next exercise step in strengthening your core and you will again utilize your yoga mat making this an exercise that you can do anywhere at any time to make sure you keep with the workout plan. To plank you will lay down with your face to the floor, then put your forearms and toes into the floor and push upwards and as you do, you will need to tighten your hip muscles, leg muscles, arm, back and chest muscles as well as your abs. The great thing about planking is that while it works your core, it also works with your other key muscles making it a full body building exercise. While you are lifted up you need to keep your entire body straight and breathe evenly for 30 seconds before you gently lower yourself back down. When you lift next you will focus on using your right side, keeping your body stacked over one another with only your right forearm and toes touching the mat, hold for 30 seconds, lower and then repeat on the left side. To create a set, you will do the trio another three to four times. As 30 seconds becomes easier you will add on another 10 seconds at a time.

The last exercise to add into your core routine is called the superman again, you will lay down on your yoga mat with your face directly facing the floor. Bring your arms in front of you and reach for the opposite side of the room. Keep your legs straight and tighten your thighs and glute muscles and then you lift your arms, chest and head up as well as your legs and feet, mimicking a superman flying pose. Keep your muscles tight and hold the pose for at least 45 seconds, then drop the pose gently and repeat. Like with the other exercises once this time period becomes easy you will increase by at least 10 seconds.

Now you are on your way to the perfect routine to get the perfect abs and get your body strengthened. You need to make sure once you start a routine for your core and general fitness that you give yourself a schedule. Give the core time to rest while you work on something else, so that you will see the top results without injuring yourself. An example of a great workout schedule includes:

- *Monday* - Strength Workout;
- *Tuesday* - Core/Ab Workout;
- *Wednesday* - Cardio Workout;
- *Thursday* - Strength Workout;
- *Friday* - Core Workout;
- *Saturday* - Cardio Workout;
- *Sunday* - Day off;

If you just have Core Workout, your schedule could be:
- *Monday* - Half an hour;
- *Tuesday* - Hour;
- *Wednesday* - Day off;
- *Thursday* - Half hour;
- *Friday* - Hour;
- *Saturday* - Day off;
- *Sunday* - Day off;

The important thing is to alternate workouts and work in a rest day. In the next chapter we will cover cardiovascular workouts.

CHAPTER 2
Basic Cardio

Cardio work is an essential exercise for your overall health and before you can understand why it is important you need to know exactly what it is. Cardiovascular fitness also known as aerobic exercise has two very distinctive features that make it different from other fitness regimes. The first is that cardio fitness will enhance your heart and lungs so that they can better supply fully oxygenated blood to all of your working muscles. The second difference is that cardio work will allow the muscles to use the oxygen that is being supplied better when the muscles are in motion.

So why is cardio important in your workout? Just looking at what cardio is, tells you exactly why it is important. You need strong lungs and a strong heart to live and when you are getting fit and working out regularly you need the extra oxygenated blood. The more oxygen you get into your blood the better your body works, it is like making sure your car has clean filters and enough mobile oil.

The great thing about a good cardio work out is that there are a great variety of exercises you can choose from so you never get bored with your exercises. While you work through this continuous activity you will be activating large muscle groups at a time and keeping them going in a steady rhythm. You must also make sure to keep your heart in a target range during some cardio work this target is found by subtracting your age from 220 and then calculating 70% to 80% of that.

Cardio exercises can include:
- Running
- Jogging
- Power walking
- Biking
- Swimming
- Dance

- Cross fit
- Cross country skiing
- Roller skating/blade

If those great options aren't enough to get you excited about cardio exercise, here are some specific exercises that are geared to get your heart and lungs going while also toning your body. Some of these are HIIT or High intensity interval training while others are basic or low intensity.

Stairmaster: This may be an oldie but it is good because it works. The Stairmaster will target your glutes and work your thighs hard, you will sweat and you will burn calories and fat. The key to how much fat you will burn and how hard the work you do on the Stairmaster is what the intensity is on the stepper. Don't get comfortable and act like you are on a simple, breezy walk on the treadmill rather make sure you are focused have the machine cranked up and put your body to work!

To get started on the Stairmaster, you will want to start with 15-35 minute sessions between two and four times a week. The best way to get the most out of your Stairmaster training is to alternate between HIIT and LISS (low intensity steady state cardio). By alternating you ensure that every muscle group gets a through work out and it will allow you to have rest days and days where you push your limit. As long as you are staying within your target heart beat range you're doing the perfect workout.

Plyometric: This cardio workout is also called Jumping Jacks-Attack and is a fast paced workout that promises not to bore you when you do it. They are a challenge to even some veterans of the workout routines, but the results they get are well worth what you go through. The good news is even through they can be tough, you can adapt them and change the movements some when you are a beginner until you get the hang of how they work.

To do this you will do as many jumping jacks as you can for 30 seconds and then rest for 30 seconds. You will then increase the time to 40 seconds and then 50 seconds. Then you will repeat this process three to four times. It may not seem like a lot, but once you get going you will feel the burn in your muscles and lungs.

Running: For some this choice may be boring but for others, running is a great way to get a solid core work out in and find stress relief as well. Those who truly love to run and train to do it often say they feel at peace when they are running and can feel their mind clear. When you go running you can put on your music and just start going down the road or down the treadmill if that is the case. The best runs will have inclines to them as you go instead of just being flat, if you are working out on the treadmill of course you can easily set the incline up and just go. The best heart healthy and fat burning regime is sprints of 20 seconds, then 45 seconds of a resting jog and repeat this cycle between 12 to 15 times. When you start to feel that these rounds aren't challenging up the sprint times and keep on going. This exercise is guaranteed to get your heart going and burn fat to help you reach a healthy place the body mass indicator scale.

Jump Rope: Take away the visions of those plastic beads covered ropes in gym class and imagine just how much you get up and moving when you start jumping rope. This is a fantastic workout to get your blood moving fast and a sweat going in a small amount of time, the best thing about jump rope is you can really tailor it to what workout you need at any given time. Are you on the road for business? Not able to get to the gym? That is okay because all you need for this is a rope. Most jumpers will set themselves to work for a set amount of time put yourself into fast sets like between 45-100 jumps in a frame of 30 seconds to a minute. Just tailor make it for yourself and get going.

These are just some of the best and easiest cardiovascular workouts that you can do to help make yourself healthier. In the next chapter we will cover HIIT in more depth and give you some hardcore workouts you can add into your HIIT schedule of exercises.

CHAPTER 3
HIIT

When you are new to body building, toning and fitness in general thinking about high-intensity interval training can be a little overwhelming but it doesn't have to be. HIIT is a hard hitting fast workout (like we briefly stated in Chapter 2) that is known to burn off a lot of calories in a short period of time. You can melt off weight and get healthy without spending hours upon hours at the gym and when you have a busy full schedule this is a great workout process. HIIT is not for everyone, if you have serious joint issues or need to focus on low impact training you do not want to do HIIT, but if you have no problem with attacking your training in bursts of full out work and then a short recovery period you are really going to enjoy the different exercises you can do with HIIT.

The first thing you need to do before a HIIT workout is warm up. You need to make sure that your muscles are limber and ready to take on the intense work you are about to put them through. Warm ups do not have to take long they just need to be thorough.

Two Minute Warm Up

Start this HIIT warm up with a simple marching in place for 30 seconds. Once you have a good marching pace going you will want to stop and stand still. One at a time lift your arms and pull them backwards in a mock swimming backstroke, this should also be done in 30 seconds. Lastly, you will do a series of lunges to get your leg muscles working, first lunge to the front, then the side than the back always using the same leg to lunge with. After 30 seconds on the first leg lunging you will switch and do another 30 seconds. Now you are warmed up and ready to go.

The Ten Minute Beginner HIIT

This workout is designed to get you going and burning off the fat while working all of your core muscle groups without any expensive gym equipment. You can do it at home, in the park anywhere you have 10 minutes of time and it is the perfect workout for those new to HIIT.

Start with your right side and put your right foot out before the left, keep your hips turned to your left side and raise your hands and up like a boxer would defend their face. Punch with your right arm, then cross punch with your left. As you throw these two punches you will move your entire body in the same motions while keeping your weight on your right foot and allowing your back foot to come off the ground a small bit. You bring both arms back in close to the body again to starting point and then you switch to your left side and do the same movements. Do this as hard as you can for 20 seconds, then rest for 10 before going into the next part of the workout.

Next come the *jumping jacks* and you will do these as fast as you can. Place your feet just hip length apart and hold your arms still at your sides until you hit the clock and start jumping out and raising your arms up in classic jumping jack style. Do as many jumping jacks as you can as fast as you can within your 20 second period then take your 10 second rest.

Sumo squats are the fourth exercise in this round of HIIT work and they promise to work your core and glutes hard! Place your feet slightly wider than hip length apart and keep your toes pointed to an angle of 45 degrees. Rock back slightly so your weight rests on your heels while your chest upright and holding tight. Lower yourself down and then push back up to the start stance by using your glutes and quads as propulsion. Once again, you will repeat this as hard and fast as you can for 20 seconds before you repeat.

Each exercise should be done in sets of three before moving on to the next and then you do the entire list three times before working in your cool down period. For cool down you will stretch your arms over your head and hold, then do a series of slow easy lunges. As you get more into your training and your fitness you will find these 10 minute training starts to get easier, that is when it is time to move your HIIT up a notch.

20 Minute HIIT

This next level of HIIT training is purposely designed to get your metabolism going and burn as many calories as possible. It will feel challenged and you might get frustrated with it the first times you work through it, but you need to stick with it and you will see the results.

This 20 minute workout has 5 different exercises that will work the whole body, joints and will be done in 45 second rounds with 15 seconds of rest.

Classic Pushups: Do as many pushups as you can in 45 seconds! If you can't do a normal pushup you can start by putting your knees on the ground in a resting position.

Squats: Squats may not be everyone's favorite, but they burn calories and work multiple muscle groups. Once again, you will do as many as you can in 45 seconds before resting. If you have trouble when you first start out you can use a chair or other stable object for support. Your feet need to remain under you and rest your weight fully on your heels.

Butt Kicks: Start jogging in place at a swift pace before you kick your leg up to touch your butt, first with your right leg and then with your left. Once again, do this rotation as many times as you can in 45 seconds, you will feel the burn in your legs and that is how you know it is working.

Tridips: Putting your arms behind you on a sturdy chair or table you will keep your back straight against the object. Next, you keep your legs straight out while you keep the weight of your body on your palms with those elbows bent, lower yourself down and then press back up. Do this process as many times as you can during your 45 seconds and don't forget to use your core muscles.

Side Lunge: Time to get your lunges back in use with this one. Your body weight should rest mostly on your heels while you keep your feet facing forward, step left and lunge down as deep as you can without letting your knee fall below your toes, come back and repeat with the right. 45 seconds of hard work with these lunges and then you rest.

Do these in sets and rotations of 3 before you do your cool down again, an overhead stretch and some basic slow moving lunges keep yourself from getting tight in the muscles!

These are the two best starter HIIT routines and once you feel comfortable with them you can change them up. Add in your own favorite workout moves and challenge yourself to go for more time. The important thing to remember when doing HIIT is that during your work time you go as hard and fast as you can no matter what the move is. Get your heart going and your muscles engaged as fast as possible.

While HIIT is fantastic not everyone can handle the high impact nature of it and that is okay. In the next chapter we will cover lower impact exercises that you can do to still get your body moving.

CHAPTER 4
Low Impact

Low impact exercise doesn't have to mean low calorie burn. In this chapter you will see how the key to having a great calorie burn without harming your knees and joins is getting the most bang for your buck in what work outs you choose, cross fit might not be right for you, but there is good calorie burning, cardio workouts that will take it easy on tender joints and make you feel great about yourself.

Walking: It may seem like walking can't do much for you to burn calories but it will burn a lot more than you think. A steady walk on a flat surface can burn between 150 and 200 calories for 45 minutes of work.

It works because when you walk you are working almost every muscle in your body. If you are just getting into working out you don't need to walk for miles on end, start with 10 minutes, then up the time every week as you work. If you feel up to really upping the burn you can start introducing more into your walk, try power walking at intervals on your walk or find an area that has slight inclines to tackle. Adding these small changes will work your muscle groups a little harder and burn more calories.

Zumba: It may sound like Zumba is just a craze, but this is a really fun low impact exercise that burns around 350 calories in 45 minutes and is guaranteed to put a smile on your face. The music is sure to get you moving and you will soon forget that you are working out, if it is your first time going to Zumba make sure you let the instructor know so they can help you make sure that your form is correct and since it is basically dance moves that are aimed at activating certain muscle groups it does not put a lot of hard work on your joints.

The Steps: You can choose to climb outdoor steps or use a climbing machine in the gym or at home, but if you work this process at a steady and even speed you will find that you can still kill calories, engage your abs and get toned without hurting yourself. While there is a HIIT exercises on the stairs as well you can keep a moderate pacing that will be low impact, try not to go above a moderate pace and when you feel tired, step away and do something else for a while, when you get tired you can become off balance and are at risk of falling off stairs or the Stairmaster.

Biking: If you love the outdoors and have a bike why not combine the two into an easy workout that will burn around 400 calories for 45 minutes of work. Keep your pace moderate and tackle the fairly flat terrain and you won't see high impact on your joints and knees as you work. If you can't get outside due to whether you can try a spin class at your local gym. Spin classes will get you moving and provide some inspiring music while you work as well. If you find you enjoy biking and spinning you can up your calorie game even more by investing in a pair of shoes designed to clip in and keep your foot at the proper angle to maximize the muscle work.

Swimming: Swimming is fantastic for cardiovascular health, but it is also the perfect work out for someone who needs to keep things low impact. If you work at a slow to moderate pace for 45 minutes when swimming you will burn around 350 calories and it can be a great deal of fun, who doesn't love being in the water? The greatest thing about doing laps is there is virtually no impact on your joints but you will build important muscle mass and burn calories while you go. When you feel yourself begin to tire takes a break at the side of the pool then go again. By allowing yourself breaks between workouts you will keep the workout going without causing damage to your joints.

As you can see there are plenty of workouts you can do that will engage your legs, back, legs, chest, shoulders and core without putting you into a place where you could do more harm than good. Any Doctor will tell patients that movement is essential, even with conditions like Rheumatoid arthritis and Fibro, it is just about finding what works the best for you.

Now that you know a wide range of workouts for every occasion it is time to find out a little bit about the fuel that you put into your body. When you start a workout program you need to look at what you eat, not just for calorie counting, but make sure your muscles have the right things to work efficiently for you.

CHAPTER 5
Fuel

What you fuel your body with while you are working to get a better place on the body mass indicator or just get in shape is as important as what workouts you do. If you don't put the right food into your body you won't get the right results when you work out. While you should seek a nutritionist for advice on building a full scale menu especially if you have large weight loss goals, there are some specific foods that are known for being healthy and great for workouts.

Oatmeal is a great way to start the day and to get your muscles ready for a workout, it is full of healthy carbs which you need during a workout. They are also full of healthy glucose, which is direct fuel for your muscles and this is a slower digesting set of carbs so you get a sustained release to your blood sugar levels, it gives you energy and makes sure you can keep going safely. Instant oatmeal works, but the top oatmeal choice is whole oats they take a little bit more time to make, but are well worth the effort as they are healthier and will digest at a slower rate.

Oysters: You may only think of these mollusks as an aphrodisiac, but they are actually jam packed with iron, which will build up your hemoglobin and make it easier for oxygen delivery throughout the body. If you skip out on iron you will start to feel it the more you work out, you will have lactic acid pumped into your muscles and it will cause you to get tired faster. If you eat as little as 6 oysters you get up to 20% of your daily value of iron for a woman and 50% for a man. That is an impressive iron for a relatively small amount of calories.

Salmon: Another great source of minerals and protein is salmon, when you eat a high quality portion of 3 ounces you will get 22 grams or more of protein which you need to ensure proper muscle growth as you work out. You get vitamin D as well, which is one that many people don't manage to get enough of in their diet and it also attributes to muscle strength and growth.

Almonds: These little nuts make a great snack, even if they seem like they are not the first thing you should grab for. When you are burning calories and working out your body produces more free radicals and they need to be dealt with before they cause too much damage. Almonds are chock full of antioxidants such as flavonoids, phenolic acids, and vitamin E these are what protects the body free radicals. Eating as little as 60 almonds per day can increase your antioxidant capacity and up your overall stamina during workouts.

Raisins: These yummy dried fruits are better for you than a sugar laden energy bar! One small box is a great fuel to get you through a workout when you feel like you may be dragging, you will find healthy carbs and potassium within them which will give you energy and help balance out your fluids, this is important if you want to stave off dehydration and muscle cramping. One small box of raisins has more potassium in it than a banana.

Water: This is a given, you need water to survive and you should be drinking more when you work out, but many forget this simple addition to their diet in favor of sports drinks and the like. Unless you have worked at a higher rate for over an hour you really don't need anything more than a healthy dose of water and you should continue to drink water throughout your day.

These are just a few of the fantastic foods that will help you. The most important thing you need to remember when you start working to tone up your core and work on your body fitness is to listen to your body. If you feel like you are missing something, you likely are if you are more tired then usual listen to that. As you lose weight and work out more it is possible you will uncover some health issues you didn't know about, get regular check ups and consult with your Doctor as you work out.

CONCLUSION

Thank you again for downloading this book!

I hope this book was able to help you to get you walking on the path to weight loss and fitness.

The next step is to put everything you have read to good use and don't forget to consult your doctor for any major changes.

REVIEW LINK

If you enjoyed this book, we would really appreciate it if you could leave us a positive REVIEW?

P.S. **You can CLICK HERE to go directly to the book page** and leave your review and/or purchase our other books above. Alternatively, you can copy and paste this address into your browser --- http://amzn.to/1wCj3OE

PREVIEW OF "CLEANSING AND DIETING BOOK BUNDLE"

Liver Cleanse and Detox Diet

The Ultimate Guide to Cleansing the Body, Eliminating Toxins and Losing Weight!

and

Anticancer Diet

The Ultimate Guide to Fighting Cancer, Lowering Risk and Achieving Optimum Health

Chapter 2

What are the Symptoms of an Unhealthy Liver?

Detection of a liver disease at an early stage is crucial to the prevention of more severe liver problems such as cirrhosis, cancer and liver failure from developing. In order to do this, you must be aware of its symptoms so that you can seek the aid of a hepatologist, a liver specialist, before anything can get really complicated. Being able to identify accurately the signs and symptoms of liver disease will greatly increase your chances of having it treated early and successfully eliminating liver disease. A very common rule of thumb, though, is to have your liver checked at least once a year.

Below is a list of signs and symptoms of an unhealthy liver, which you can easily identify. Practically, these are symptoms you can detect on your own and without any aid of a professional doctor or a hepatologist. However, if you suspect that you have liver disease based on your personal assessment according to the signs and symptoms you've learned here, it is always best to consult with your physician. Do not consider this list as completely conclusive.

Common Signs of an Unhealthy Liver

There's a myriad of liver diseases and the symptoms may tend to be specific for that particular kind of illness until the later stage of liver disease or worse, when liver failure occurs.

The initial symptoms are signs that can also happen and be caused by other problems in the body, making it rather difficult to identify liver diseases with certainty. These symptoms include nausea and vomiting, loss of appetite, diarrhea and fatigue or the feeling of being weak.

However, with the lack of immediate medication and as the complication progresses, the symptoms become more serious and require immediate care. These signs include:

Abdominal Pain

This may be the result of having gallstones, the most common is cholesterol gallstones, which can be found usually deposited in the gallbladder and bile ducts. Pain is experienced in the upper right abdominal area of the body, and fever may occur when there is an infection in the gallbladder as a result of this.

Jaundice

This is a condition wherein there is too much bilirubin in the bloodstream. Bilirubin is mainly processed in the liver, therefore this excess that turns the skin, eyes and the mucus membranes in the mouth to turn yellow indicates liver damage, which can lead to liver failure if the cause is not treated.

Extreme Sleepiness

As cirrhosis, an advanced liver disease caused by a scar tissue in an attempt to perform the repair of damaged tissues by the liver, develops it causes further complications. One of these complications is called hepatic encephalopathy, which stops the liver from getting the blood clear of ammonia and other nitrogenous substances, affecting the cerebral functioning, such as forgetfulness, unresponsiveness, inability to concentrate and extreme sleepiness even during daytime, when it is carried to the brain.

Weight loss

A sudden decrease in weight can be caused by more than several factors. Loss of appetite, persistent vomiting, malabsorption and increased metabolism can be some of the most obvious causes. However, there's also some evidence that points to systemic diseases such as liver diseases as one of its causes.

If you like this preview, then *click here for the full story of this eBook!*

Or go to: *http://www.amazon.com/dp/B00QX9ENDC/*

ANTICANCER DIET

The Ultimate Guide to Fighting Cancer, Lowering Risk and Achieving Optimum Health

Chapter 2
Preventing Cancer through Diet

True to the famous cliché, "Prevention is better than cure", there are natural ways to prevent the risk of having a cancer. One of which is through healthy living and diet. Every person must consider eating a healthy diet regardless of family history related to cancer. Diet makes a major difference in the battle of this disease by increasing immunity.

Connection between Diet and Cancer

It is evident, there are many unavoidable health problems, however, you have major control over your own health, far more than you can imagine. Lifestyle choices affect the way cancer cells develop. A large percentage of deaths related to cancer root from lifestyle choices. Avoiding vices and addictions will surely help in staying healthy.

The foods that you eat and the ones you avoid having a powerful impact on your health. Unknown to you, you might be gradually fueling the cancer- cell production process through the food that you are eating. You should not ignore the nutrients and benefits that your diet might bring. Minimization of risks will be highly regarded by your discipline in diet.

Maintain a Healthy Weight

The best way to obtain your healthy weight is by conducting a test of Body Mass Index or BMI. This is the ratio between your weight and height. The need to reduce the risk of cancer gives a person a margin up to the score of 25. If you cannot comprehend the implication of your BMI, you can consult your doctor and seek an advice.

Moreover, maintaining a healthy weight reduces the tendency of complications such as diabetes and heart disease. If you are obese, you are prone to some types of cancer, such as colon, endometrium, breast, pancreas, esophagus and kidney. Also, excessive weight can aid in producing and circulating insulin and estrogen, which can stimulate the production of cancer-producing cells.

If you like this preview, then *click here for the full story of this eBook!*

Or go to: *http://www.amazon.com/dp/B00QXO08oE/*

CHECK OUT MY OTHER BOOKS

Teeth Healing through Oil Pulling

The Complete Guide in Natural Oral Care through the Benefits of Oil Pulling

10 Things You Need to Know about Ebola

Facts about the Virus, Symptoms, Quarantine and Prevention

Paleo and Grain-Free Diet for Beginners

Cookbook Recipes using a Slow Cooker for Weight Loss

Gout Cure

Your Ultimate and Comprehensive Guide in Treating Gout Permanently

Mediterranean Diet for Beginners

Cuisine Cookbook Recipes for Shredding Fat and Weight Loss

Slimming Secrets

Health, Fitness, and Diet Secrets for the New You

DEDICATION

To our three blessings that have made RicTamily complete and continue to grow together in His loving embrace.

DISCLAIMER

The information in this book is in no way intended as medical advice. This book is not meant to be used, nor should it be used, to diagnose or treat any medical condition. The author disclaims responsibility for any adverse health effects that come in combination with the use of methods and suggestions presented in the book. The publisher and author are not responsible for any health or allergy needs that may require medical supervision and are not liable for any damages or negative consequences from any treatment, action, application or preparation, to any person reading or following the information in this book.